EATING ON-THE-GO

The Traveler's Guide to Healthy Eating

Master this knowledge as if your life
depends on it…because it does!

ROXANNE EDRINGTON

INTRODUCTION

If you're someone who travels, and you struggle to eat healthy on-the-go, this book is for you! No more excuses -- the time is now! Research has shown "If you ask an adult in the later years of their life what they value most, **"good health"** is at the top of their list. Prolonging life without prolonging the "quality" of life is not the goal for most people. People are looking for ways to "add life" to their years and not years to their life." Traveling and living on the road has a huge impact on our health. Sleeping in different beds, skipping meals, eating whatever and whenever we can...all attribute to unhealthy aging. Although we tend to get caught up in this never ending merry-go-round, the good news is the healthy choices we make today will impact our health in the future. I believe with some education, everyone can stop the madness and eat for success.

If you're looking for ways to eat healthy while on the road, I have the solution! I'm a clinical nutritionist, chiropractor, lifestyle coach, public speaker, athlete and a mother of two with numerous titles in the Health and Fitness world including: Ms. World Cup, Ms. Texas and Ms. Southern States. I've run marathons, and played on The Houston Energy, a women's professional football team in which I acquired several SuperBowl rings. I entered my first triathlon in 2012 and competed in Ironman Florida and Ironman Texas in 2015 and 2016. Shortly after, I competed on American Ninja Warrior and I currently still compete in ninja competitions. If ANYONE needed to come up with a plan to eat-on-the-go...it was ME! Not only because I am EXTREMELY busy and I travel a lot; but, because my family history is saturated with obesity, diabetes, heart disease and cancer. I knew if I didn't master eating on-the-go, my chances of becoming plagued with a chronic illness were extremely high.

The #1 obstacle I see with my patients who travel is "eating on-the-go." Most of them do well with their eating plan at home, but as soon as they pack their bags and head out the door...the wheels fall off. Their biggest struggle? They don't know what to eat -- or what to order -- when they're on the road. After years of practice, I've found a solution that works.

Meet David, a 42-year old executive that entered the corporate world five years ago. When he began, David was a healthy, energetic and outgoing guy. His new job required a lot of travel, however, and he came to my office complaining of low energy and weight gain. His diagnosis? David had high cholesterol, high blood pressure and was pre-diabetic.

This is a common scenario…I see it every day in my practice. Once I drilled down into David's life, I realized his health problems were the result of food choices he'd made while eating on-the-go. Once he implemented the strategies outlined in this book, David lost weight, had an enormous amount of energy and his lab values normalized.

You, too, can learn how to eat on-the-go so you can prevent - or even reverse your chances for developing - a chronic illness. So what are you waiting for? Let's begin the journey!

TABLE OF CONTENTS

CHAPTER ONE

HOW SHOULD YOU EAT?

Scientific research is proving that living a healthy lifestyle reduces premature disability and chronic illnesses experienced by many people. But, it's a simple fact that life has become more hectic, and, as a result, we rely on highly processed convenience foods. By sacrificing nutrition for ease and accessibility, we're ignoring the long-term consequences to our health. Dependence on these high-fat, high-sugar "junk foods" has caused a rise in the occurrence of hypertension, heart disease, diabetes, high cholesterol and obesity in both adults and children.

So what can we do?

One of the biggest problems is that for every question we have, there are many opposing answers. We're all on information overload – "googled out," so to speak. So how do we distinguish good from bad advice?

1

In this chapter, I'll teach you how to eat for success. By following these principles you'll be able to make simple changes in your eating plan to be healthy and have more energy. People who have followed these basic guidelines feel fantastic! So let's get started.

BALANCED BLOOD SUGAR

The basic principal for success is keeping your blood sugar BALANCED throughout the day. This is the key to having more energy, improving your health and becoming a fat burning machine. It's natural for our energy levels to fluctuate throughout the day. When we wake up in the morning we want to feel energetic and before we go to bed at night we want to feel sleepy. What about the rest of the day? How you feel during the day has EVERYTHING to do with your management of food. The way you eat will affect your mental clarity, your concentration, your productivity and your sense of well-being.

Signs and Symptoms of "_Unbalanced_" Blood Sugar Levels:

- Fatigue/sleepy
- Inability to concentrate
- Depressed
- Irritable
- Mood swings

- Unmotivated
- No energy at the end of the day to do chores or exercise
- Food cravings - especially for sugar or carbohydrates
- Body is more prone to store fat

Signs and Symptoms of "_Balanced_" Blood Sugar Levels:

- Increased energy
- Motivated
- Better ability to focus
- Increased mental clarity
- Increased memory
- No food or sugar cravings
- No mood swings
- Increased self confidence
- Body is more prone to burn fat

It's important to understand how your body manages your food intake. Seemingly harmless little habits can be zapping your energy. Almost everything you eat or drink is digested and broken down to a sugar called **glucose**. Glucose is the type of sugar found in your blood and it is "the sugar" you are trying to balance. All the cells in your body require a steady supply of glucose for energy. _Too much_ or _too_ *little* glucose in your blood stream is not good. Both contribute to unbalanced blood sugar.

So, how do you maintain *balanced* blood sugar levels throughout the day?

1. Consume Low Glycemic Index (GI) foods
2. Eat smaller meals more frequently

LOW GLYCEMIC INDEX FOODS

The most successful way to keep your blood sugar balanced throughout the day is by eating low glycemic index (GI) foods. What is the glycemic index of food? It's the measure of *the rate* at which ingested food causes glucose levels to rise in the blood.

High GI foods: The glycemic index value is 70 or greater

Medium (GI) foods: The glycemic index value is 56 to 69

Low (GI) foods: The glycemic index value is 55 and below

High GI foods break down into glucose very quickly. You can distinguish these foods by putting them into a bowl and adding water. Any food that gets soggy or dissolves within 1-3 minutes when liquid is added (i.e., cereal, bread, crackers, chips etc) is a high GI food. These foods "dump" glucose into the system rapidly causing a spike in insulin resulting in fat storage.

Conversely, low GI foods break down into glucose much more slowly. These foods typically do not get soggy or dissolve when submerged in water. Examples of low GI foods are proteins, oils, fats, most vegetables and certain grains and fruits. These foods "drip" glucose into the system helping the body maintain balanced blood sugar levels.

MEAL FREQUENCY

The second key to maintaining balanced blood sugar levels is meal frequency. WHAT you eat is important, but equally important in balancing your blood sugar levels is WHEN you eat. It's the slow rise and fall in blood sugar levels throughout the day that enables your brain and body to work and play with good energy. Each meal should consist of approximately 250 to 400 calories of low GI foods depending on your gender and activity level. When the body is able to use all the sugar that is dripping slowly, steadily and continuously into the system as fuel to perform cellular functions, nothing is being stored as fat. Your energy doesn't spike and drop throughout the day. You feel great! What's more, you've turned your body into an efficient, fat-burning machine.

Let me explain this to you in more detail. It takes approximately 2 1/2 to 3 hours to utilize the glucose in low GI foods. When you eat a chicken breast and vegetables, it slowly digests into glucose. Your cells will steadily use up all the glucose with a minimal rise in blood sugar, leaving no excess to be stored. Two and a half hours later, however, unless you eat another low GI snack, your blood sugar levels start to drop. You've avoided the "ups" but not the "downs." This drop in blood sugar will create mood swings, fatigue, and cravings that will send you racing to the vending machine. At this point, you won't care about choosing a low GI food so your derailment begins. You decide to eat whatever is convenient. Soon, your blood sugar level spikes, due to high amounts of insulin secreted which will lead to an unhealthy chain of events including low energy and poor mental clarity. So eat low GI foods every three hours to keep your blood sugar balanced!

So what does all of this mean? Eat many small meals comprised of low GI foods throughout the day. Do not exceed the 3 hour mark. This will eliminate your worst enemy... **HUNGER**. It you skip meals, or wait until you're hungry to eat...IT'S OVER!! The executive centers inside the brain begin chanting "Feed me! Feed me!" and you will crave a high fat, high sugar meal and start the process all over! This doesn't mean you're not disciplined or that you're a weak individual. What it means is that your brain needs glucose, and simple sugars and carbohydrates are the fastest way to get glucose into the system. Remember, we don't want to "dump" glucose into the system. If we do, we'll become a fat-depositing machine. This is what happens when we eat high GI foods. We want to eat low GI foods that "drip" glucose into our system so that we become a fat-burning machine!

In the Appendix, there is a list of which foods you should INCLUDE and which foods you should AVOID in your meal planning decisions. I have also included a sample menu guide in Chapter 2. This will help you make better choices while you are eating on-the-go.

KEY POINTS:

- · Keeping your blood sugar balanced throughout the day is the key to having more energy, improved health and a faster metabolism.
- · The two ways to balance your blood sugar: eat low glycemic index (GI) foods and eat 5-6 mini-meals throughout the day.

CHAPTER TWO

WHAT ARE GOOD FOOD CHOICES?

Every day I have a new patient walk into my office and tell me their diet is "almost perfect" but they still don't feel well. They are NOT coming to see me for advice on their food intake; they are coming to see me about a possible nutrient deficiency. Meet Dorothy, a successful, intelligent mother of two. She's an avid reader and very knowledgeable on health and fitness topics. She trains with a trainer twice a week and feels like she's mastered her eating plan. After I listened to her story and her concerns, we went over her daily meal plan. I was astonished by some of her food choices! When I asked her about these choices, she said, "I read somewhere that new research has shown that it's good for my health – even the label said it.?

One of the biggest problems I see is that people believe what they read on food labels. I know that sounds logical but don't do it. The food industry has found ways to have us believe certain foods are "healthy." How do they do it? Remember, the food industry is a multi-billion dollar industry whose main goal is to sell products. These corporations devise great marketing strategies to draw your money into their pockets. If eating healthy is your goal…you'll find all kinds of catch phrases on food labels to get you to buy their product.

So, what should you eat? Again, focus on eating a balance of low GI foods throughout the day. If you can memorize good food choices from the Food List in the Appendix, and learn how to put them together to make a balanced meal, you'll be able to eat for success.

MENU GUIDES

The guides on the following pages show you how to plan your day with meals for success. Some people may have different philosophies on eating fats or starches. This is perfectly ok. You can substitute a fat for a carbohydrate or visa versa. I have worked with all diets and this meal plan has worked best. I realize you won't always be able to follow this template perfectly, but it will help you make better decisions when ordering meals. Sample menus also are included.

DAILY MENU GUIDE FOR MEN

FOOD LIST is in the Appendix

BREAKFAST 6:00	Protein source 1 starch/grain OR 1 serving of fat
SNACK 9:00	Low GI snack or protein shake
LUNCH 12:00	6 oz. of lean meat (review Food List) 1 c of vegetables/salad (review Food List) 1 starch/grain OR 1 serving of fat
SNACK 3:00	Low GI snack or protein shake
DINNER 6:00	6 oz. of lean meat (review Food List) 1 cup of vegetables/salad (review Food List) 1 starch/grain OR 1 serving of fat
SNACK	Low GI snack or 7-8 natural nuts

* Examples of starches/grains

- 3/4 cup of Kashi GOLEAN Cereal or Hi-Lo Cereal
- 3/4 cup rice or 3/4 cup pasta
- 6 oz potato
- 2-3 corn tortillas
- ½ cup beans

SAMPLE MENU #1 FOR MEN

BREAKFAST Choose one	6 egg whites scrambled with seasonings and 1/2 cup slow cooked oatmeal 6 egg whites omelet with onions, mushrooms and tomatoes with avocado 2/3 cup of egg substitute scrambled with bell peppers, onions in 2 corn tortillas Protein shake
SNACK Choose one	1 piece of fruit and 1 serving of nuts 1 serving of nuts 3-6 oz. of chicken salad or tuna salad
LUNCH Choose one	2 cups spinach salad with 6 oz of fish, chicken breast, shrimp or scallops 1/4 avocado and slivered almonds 6 oz of fish, chicken breast, shrimp or scallops; steamed veggies and rice or baked potato 6 oz chicken breast or fish with 1 cup steamed broccoli
SNACK Choose one	Protein shake 1 serving of nuts 1/2 cup hummus with veggies 1 cup chicken salad or tuna fish salad

DINNER Choose one	Mixed greens with 6 oz chicken breast, fish or shrimp 6 oz sea bass with 1 cup of steamed asparagus and rice or a baked potato
SNACK Choose one	Boiled eggs 1/2 cup blueberries and 8-10 walnuts, almonds or pecans

SAMPLE MENU #2 FOR MEN

BREAKFAST Choose one	6 egg whites scrambled with onions, mushrooms, spinach, tomatoes and salsa rolled up in 2 corn tortillas 1 cup Kashi *GOLEAN* cereal with a pinch of slivered almonds Egg white omelet with veggies topped with goat cheese
SNACK Choose one	1 piece of fruit (review the Food List) and 8 almonds or walnuts Protein shake

LUNCH Choose one	2 cups spinach salad with 6 oz chicken breast, 1/4 avocado and ½ cup of chick-peas Chicken fajitas with salsa, beans and avocado and 2-3 corn tortillas 6 oz chicken breast or fish with ¾ cup rice and 1 cup veggies
SNACK Choose one	Protein shake 1 apple and 8-10 walnuts, almonds or pecans
DINNER Choose one	6 oz. of tuna steak with fresh lemon juice, 1 cup of rice steamed spinach 6 oz lean beef, 6 oz sweet potato and 1 cup of steamed broccoli or veggies Two cups of tossed salad with 6 oz of grilled chicken breast
SNACK Choose one	Nonfat Greek yogurt with added fruit 4 egg white omelet topped with salsa

DAILY MENU GUIDE FOR WOMEN

FOOD LIST is in the Appendix

BREAKFAST 6:00	Protein source 1 starch/grain OR 1 serving of fat
SNACK 9:00	Low GI snack or protein shake
LUNCH 12:00	4 oz of lean meat (review Food List) 1 cup of vegetables (review Food List) 1 starch/grain OR 1 serving of fat
SNACK 3:00	Low GI snack or protein shake
DINNER 6:00	4 oz of lean meat (review Food List) 1 cup of vegetables (review Food List) 1 starch/grain (optional) OR 1 serving of fat
SNACK 9:00	Low GI snack or 7 – 10 nuts (review Food List)

*Examples of starches/grains

- ½ cup of Kashi GOLEAN Cereal or Hi-Lo Cereal
- 1/4-1/2 cup rice or ½ cup pasta
- 4 oz potato
- 1-2 corn tortillas
- ½ cup beans

SAMPLE MENU #1 FOR WOMEN

BREAKFAST Choose one	4 egg whites scrambled with seasonings and 1/2 cup slow cooked oatmeal 4 egg whites omelet with onions, mushrooms, tomatoes and feta cheese 2/3 cup of egg substitute scrambled with bell peppers, onions and avocado (1-2 corn tortillas optional) Protein shake
SNACK Choose one	1 piece of fruit (review Food List) and 1 serving of nuts 1 serving of nuts (review Food List) 3-4 oz. of chicken salad or tuna salad
LUNCH Choose one	2 cups spinach salad with 4 oz of fish, chicken breast, shrimp or scallops 1/4 avocado 1 cup chicken salad or tuna fish salad (put on 6 crackers) 4 oz chicken breast or fish with 1 cup steamed broccoli
SNACK Choose one	Protein shake 1 serving of nuts 1/4 cup hummus with veggies 4 oz. chicken salad or tuna fish salad

DINNER Choose one	Mixed greens with 4 oz chicken breast or fish 4 oz sea bass with 1 cup of steamed asparagus
SNACK Choose one	2 boiled eggs 7-10 almonds or walnuts

SAMPLE MENU #2 FOR WOMEN

BREAKFAST Choose one	4 egg whites scrambled with onions, mushrooms, spinach, tomatoes and salsa rolled up in 2 corn tortillas 1 cup Kashi *GOLEAN* cereal with a pinch of slivered almonds Egg white omelet with veggies topped with fat free cheese
SNACK Choose one	4 boiled egg whites 3 oz. of chicken/tuna salad
LUNCH Choose one	2 cups spinach salad with 4 oz chicken breast, 1/4 avocado Chicken fajitas with salsa, beans and avocado and 2 corn tortillas 4 oz chicken breast or fish with ½ cup c rice and 1 cup veggies

SNACK Choose one	Protein shake 1 apple and 8-10 walnuts, almonds or pecans
DINNER Choose one	4 oz of tuna steak with fresh lemon juice, 1/2 cup of rice and steamed spinach 4 oz lean beef, 4 oz sweet potato and 1 cup of steamed broccoli or veggies Two cups of tossed salad with 4 oz of grilled chicken breast
SNACK Choose one	Nonfat Greek yogurt with added fruit 4 egg white omelet topped with salsa

CHAPTER 3

WHAT IF YOU'RE ALWAYS ON THE ROAD?

If you read one chapter of this book — read this one. Master it. It includes my three keys for successful eating on-the-go, and will give you detailed information on making healthy choices when traveling.

You *can* eat right – even if you're always on the road. Meet Gary, a successful business owner who travels extensively. He jumps into his car early in the morning and doesn't stop until he needs to fill his gas tank. When he arrives at the gas station he's hungry so he grabs a pastry or a doughnut, a banana and a coke or cup of coffee. He feels pretty good for the first hour but then starts to feel really tired. He stops again, at another food place, thinking a candy bar - or some type of fast food - will help give him more energy. Throughout the entire day, he feels sluggish, fatigued and out of sorts. Gary thinks it's because he is traveling. What he doesn't know is that it's NOT because he is traveling…he feels bad because of his food choices and meal planning while eating-on-the-go! This was a concern of Gary's because diabetes runs in his family. After Gary understood WHAT he needed to do and HOW he could implement these changes, he began to feel fantastic and even lost some unwanted weight! Gary just needed some instruction on how to eat on-the-go while he was traveling.

I know I've said this before, but I can't stress enough that the single, most important concept to remember while on the road is to eat low GI foods frequently - every 2 1/2 to 3 hours. If you wait until you're hungry…it's over! We all know what it's like to walk into a gas station or convenience store and just grab the first food that appeals to us. But, if you learn the "balancing" act, and learn it well, you won't feel exhausted and crave the wrong types of foods.

There are three things you can do to have a successful road trip of eating-on-the-go: **plan, prepare** and **pack** your food prior to leaving. There will be some of you who DO NOT want to go through the "hassle" of preparing. If this is you, skip down to the section on **"What if I don't have the time to plan, prepare or pack?"** and follow the suggested guidelines.

PLANNING

To be successful, PLAN AHEAD. Get a game plan going focused on what you need to do to make your road trip successful. Are you planning to travel with snack items but stop at food places to eat breakfast, lunch and dinner? Or, do you want to prepare food and take it with you on the road so you have more control over what you eat? Either way, take some time and contemplate how you'll meet your goals. Remember, **if you fail to plan, you are planning to fail!** It is as simple as that. In the Appendix I have included a food journal. You can use this journal to plan your meals or to keep track of the meals you're eating throughout the week.

The most challenging part of this process is getting organized. In the beginning, this might seem a little overwhelming, but after you've gone through this process a couple of times, you'll find it's not only very rewarding, but worth the extra hassle. To plan for your success, you will want to review the Dr. Roxanne approved "**Food List.**" Next, put a grocery list together of foods and other items you might need for your trip. Here is an example of **my shopping list:**

· Rotisserie chicken
· Chicken breast in a can (in water)
· Tuna fish in a can (in water)
· Boiled eggs

- Fruit from the Food List
- Veggies (in the produce section you can find veggies already cut up and ready to eat)
- Guacamole in snack size packages
- Nonfat plain Greek yogurt
- Whole grain bread with nuts and seeds
- Turkey jerky
- Protein powder (I buy Vanilla Egg White protein powder that is low in carbohydrates. By low I mean less than 10 grams)
- Natural almonds, walnuts or pecans (The only ingredient is the nut. Some may have salt added. That is ok)
- Almond milk (for my protein shakes)
- Water
- A cooler for my food
- A shaker cup for my protein drinks

PREPARING

It's IMPERATIVE to prepare your balanced meals or snacks *in advance* so you'll have food available on the fly! Review the Meal Plan from Chapter Two and get acquainted with the Sample Menus so you can prepare and plan out your meals accordingly. Make sure you write down the time you plan to eat each meal or snack. This will ensure that you don't just "wing it" and you are eating at specific times to keep your blood sugar balanced.

If you have time, make some balanced meals and put them in Tupperware containers a day or so before you leave. You can heat these meals up in a microwave on the road. Almost all convenience stores or gas stations have a microwave. As long as you buy something in the store, they don't seem to mind if you use their microwave. Here are some ideas:

· Grill or bake some lean beef, chicken or fish
· Cook some vegetables from the Food List
· Cook some rice or baked potatoes
· Boil a dozen eggs
· Make homemade chicken salad or use chicken breast in a can to speed up the process
· Prepare tuna salad from a can
· Cut up veggies to eat as a snack
· Put nuts in snack-sized baggies
· Place one serving of protein powder in several baggies

Another option is to buy healthy meals that are already prepared. In Houston, there are several establishments that offer healthy prepared meals. Go online and google "healthy prepared meals" in your area. There are also companies that deliver meals to your home. I use Livingplate.org. This is a convenient way to have food available when it's time to eat. When I know I'll be on the road for a couple of days, I stop by the store and grab several different breakfasts, lunches and dinners. By doing this, I know I have healthy food available when I need it. It eliminates any drama!

If you do plan to eat out for breakfast, lunch and dinner, or you **don't have time to prepare any meals**, focus on preparing snack foods. Chicken, tuna and egg salad are great options. I make a big bowl of it, place it in Tupperware containers, and use it as a dip for vegetables like celery, carrots, broccoli and cucumbers. Sometimes I eat it on crackers. Other times I put it on one piece of multi-grain bread. Here are my recipes:

Chicken or Tuna Salad:

· Take 2-6 large cans of tuna fish or chicken breast and put them in a bowl
· Chop one apple, several celery stalks and 1/4 cup of onions
· Scramble 6 egg whites in a skillet on the stove
· Add a small amount of dill relish (optional)
· Combine all the ingredients together in a bowl

- Sprinkle 1 tsp of dill weed seasoning to the mix
- Add a small amount of fat free mayonnaise or mustard

Stir all the ingredients together and refrigerate.

Egg Salad:

- 12 hard boiled eggs
- 4 Tbsp. mustard
- 1 Tbsp. fat free mayo
- Dill weed seasoning
- 1-2 Tbsp dill relish

SNACK IDEAS

1. If you like boiled eggs, make some boiled eggs. As a snack, they're a great way to keep your blood sugar balanced. If you're concerned about cholesterol, dump out most of the yolk and eat the egg whites only. (The white part of the egg is where all the protein is.) I typically eat 4 egg whites for a snack. Sprinkle your favorite seasoning on the egg to give it flavor or dump out the yellow and put chicken salad, hummus or guacamole in its place.

2. Cut up veggies from the Food List and place them in several zip-lock baggies. I think about how many veggies I would want to eat at a time and put that

amount in each baggie. This makes it convenient to grab a baggie and eat them on the road.

3. Similarly, cut up fresh fruit from the Food List and place it in several zip-lock baggies. Look at the serving size for each fruit and put that amount in each baggie.

4. Organize the nuts into serving sizes and place them in several snack size baggies. Each baggie should have about 10-12 nuts. By placing them in the baggies, you will be eliminating the possibility of mindless eating. Nuts are almost like potato chips…once you start eating them, it's hard to stop.

5. Grab the protein powder and place one serving in several zip-locked baggies. By doing this, you won't have to hassle with the container or scooper. You can just grab a baggie of protein powder and dump it directly into the shaker cup of water or an alternative beverage.

6. Take several containers of nonfat plain Greek yogurt. If you want to add flavor to the yogurt, put in some fruit from the Food List.

PACKING

Now just bring it all together. Place all the food you prepared in a cooler – your fruit, yogurt, protein powder and other healthy items. Don't forget to pack utensils and paper towels.

WHAT IF YOU DON'T HAVE TIME TO PLAN, PREPARE OR PACK?

There will be times you don't have the luxury to plan, prepare and pack. In fact, I've seen people who prefer to "figure it out" along the way. If this is you…no sweat. You can still eat healthy on-the-go as long as you have something available to eat every 3 hours. Stop at a store and pick up some healthy snacks Look at the list above for some snack ideas.

If you're not very hungry while traveling, try to stay on your meal frequency schedule anyway. Order a meal and eat half of it now and eat the other half a couple of hours later for a snack. This will keep your blood sugar balanced and you will have more energy and less fatigue.

Breakfast On-the-Go

FASTFOOD OPTIONS:
- Breakfast wrap or breakfast taco without cheese
- Scramble eggs with a side of fruit

GAS STATION or CONVENIENCE STORE:
- Fruit
- 1 oz. almonds, walnuts, pecans or cashews

· Nonfat plain Greek yogurt

· Water for protein shake

RESTAURANT OPTIONS: Refer to Chapter Four for restaurant ideas.

Lunch and Dinner On-the-Go

FAST FOOD OPTIONS:

Hamburger place

1. Grilled chicken sandwich with veggies (lettuce, tomatoes, pickles and onions). No mayo. Take one of the buns off to decrease carb intake. Order a side of fruit.

2. Baked potato- some places have baked potatoes. Order it dry and order a grilled chicken breast. Cut up the chicken breast and add it as a topping on the potato.

3. Grilled chicken breast salad. Order your salad with fat free dressing.

4. Grilled chicken wrap - no mayo or cheese.

Mexican place

1. Two soft tacos with chicken fajita meat and veggies. Add guacamole or hot sauce for flavor.

2. Chicken fajita taco salad. Use hot sauce of pico de gallo for the salad dressing.

Chinese place

1. Steamed chicken with steamed veggies and steamed rice. Use lite soy sauce or hot mustard for flavoring.

2. Steamed seafood with mixed vegetables and steamed rice.

Chicken place

1. Grilled chicken breast with no skin. Side of veggies or fruit.

2. Grilled chicken sandwich. No mayo. Side of fruit or veggies.

3. Grilled chicken salad. Use fat free dressing.

4. Grilled chicken wrap - no mayo or cheese.

BBQ place

1. Grilled chicken breast with pickles and onions and a small amount of BBQ sauce

2. Grilled chicken breast with a dry baked potato. Cut up the chicken and place it in the dry baked potato with a small amount of BBQ sauce. If the baked potato is HUGE… only eat half of the potato and save the rest for another meal.

Sandwich place

1. Grilled chicken breast sandwich- real chicken breast... no deli meat if possible. Add lots of veggies and avocado for flavor. If you are watching your carbohydrate intake, take off the top piece of bread.

2. Turkey or chicken breast sandwich. Double the meat. Load it up with veggies and omit mayo and cheese. If you are watching your carbohydrate intake, take off the top piece of bread.

3. Grilled chicken wraps. Load it up with veggies and omit mayo and cheese.

4. Grilled chicken breast salad. Use fat free dressing.

GAS STATIONS and CONVENIENCE STORE OPTIONS:

1. Tuna kit (in water) or Chicken breast in a can. Have an apple and 10-12 nuts.

2. Water for a protein shake and a piece of fruit.

3. Turkey jerky and some nuts

RESTAURANT OPTIONS: Refer to Chapter Four for restaurant ideas.

Remember, it's important to eat a meal or snack every 2 1/2 to 3 hours. I know when you're on the road this may seem impossible, but the results are well worth the hassle.

KEY POINTS:

- Plan ahead. Determine what you will need for your trip to make it successful.

- Stop by the grocery store prior to your trip. Pick up some items so you will have food accessible while you are on the road.

- Remember to eat something every 2 1/2 -3 hours. This will keep your blood sugar balanced which will improve your energy and well-being while traveling.

- Take a cooler to keep your food cool. This can be a collapsible lunch bag or a large cooler, depending on how much food you decide to take.

- Follow the Dr. Roxanne's approved Food List in the Appendix when ordering and buying food.

- Refer to the Menu Plan and Sample Menu Plan in Chapter Two for guidance on portion sizes and meal options.

CHAPTER FOUR

WHAT IF YOU EAT OUT AT RESTAURANTS?

The #1 obstacle I see with travelers trying to eat healthy is eating on-the-go at restaurants. By the time they arrive they're famished. They don't care about making the right choice, they just want food. They eat the basket of bread on the table and ask for a second basket. They want food and they want it NOW! And, there are so many conflicting suggestions out there on how to eat that it's difficult to make a decision. As soon as they walk into a restaurant, they are CONFUSED about what to order. Most just open the menu and order like the rest of the group. They overeat and then leave the restaurant feeling stuffed and miserable. The next day they wake up and it starts all over again! If this was only ONE meal a week, that would be ok. The problem is that it happens three times a day for a week. The consequences for this type of lifestyle can be serious – many become a high blood pressure, high cholesterol or diabetic statistic! Don't let this be you.

I travel ALL the time and I find it very easy to order healthy food while eating-on-the-go. The secret is to **prepare** your mind, **plan** ahead and be **assertive**. Many fine restaurants are extremely accommodating to the health-conscious public. Once you understand some of the basic principles, it's quite easy.

The most important thing you need to do is **ANTICIPATE ALL** possible obstacles before you get to the restaurant. Get yourself in the proper state of mind and plan what you're going to eat before you walk in.

HOW DO YOU ORDER YOUR FOOD?

When you get to the restaurant, DO NOT take a menu. Don't even open it. This will eliminate any temptation of making a poor choice and it will make a clear statement to your server that you are ordering something OFF the menu. Tell your server what YOU wish to order. I usually order ahi tuna or sea bass with steamed asparagus. If I'm really hungry I'll order a baked or sweet potato dry with the toppings on the side. In my experience, the server is very accommodating and happy to help. Even if it's not on the menu, most of the time they will prepare your meal just the way you want it.

Remember, restaurants are competing for your business. They're looking for ways to make their food taste better - not for the benefit of your health but hoping you'll return. When ordering, ask that your meal be prepared without the customary marinade, oil, butter, etc. Insist that your protein source be grilled, baked or pan-seared with fat-free cooking spray. Customarily, restaurants will have steamed vegetables. Request that no oil or butter be used on the vegetables. Other condiments such as herbs and spices are recommended to enhance flavor. Order steamed rice or a small baked potato for your carbohydrate intake. Ask for your potato to be dry with toppings on the side. If you were dining with me, this is what you would hear me tell my server:

"Hi. May I have a house salad without cheese and Balsamic Vinegar on the side. For my entrée I would like the sea bass steamed, with no butter or oil and put any toppings on the side. Do you have steamed asparagus or broccoli? I would like the steamed asparagus with no oil or butter. Do you have sweet potatoes? May I have a sweet potato with everything on the side? Please bring some ketchup.(Sometimes I put a little ketchup on my dry potato). Thank you."

That is basically my dialogue for chicken, a fillet of beef or fish. If you're watching your carbohydrate intake, order a salad instead of rice or baked potato. When ordering a salad, ask the server to place the salad dressing on the side. I usually get fat-free French, fat-free Italian or Balsamic Vinegar. It's your preference whether or not to pour the dressing onto the salad, or dip the salad into the dressing. I occasionally will take my own salad dressing into the restaurant. Salad dressings are extremely high in calories and in fat. By taking my own, I'm assured to have a low fat and healthy salad.

OK... you did a great job on ordering your food, but what do you do about the bread or chips that are brought to your table? (That was so rude of the waiter!) Believe it or not, ordering HOT tea or coffee at the beginning of a meal typically decreases cravings to eat the bread or chips placed in front of you. I have used this trick 1,000 times and it always works! The other option is to request that these items NOT be brought to the table or place those "tempting" items on the opposite side of the table.

Once your meal arrives, take small bites and be sure to chew your food at least 20 times before swallowing. Take your time, drink water and enjoy your "dining out" experience. You may not feel COMPETELY full when you have completed your meal. DO NOT WORRY. After your meal, once again, order something hot to drink. This will increase your satiety and decrease your craving for something sweet.

When it comes time for dessert, please...really? If you have followed the above referenced tips, you will have that "satisfied" feeling, I promise! On the occasion that you just WANT dessert, even if you are full, order some fresh fruit or take a couple of bites from someone else's dessert. This way you won't feel deprived.

HOW DO YOU MAINTAIN CONTROL?

There are a couple of things you can do to help with hunger and cravings. I touched on one of the methods in the paragraph above. I call it the "hot tea/coffee" trick. Often, after I eat, I still feel hungry and/or I crave something sweet. I eat frequently, so I know it's not because I'm depriving myself. So here is a little trick: After I eat a meal or a snack, I immediately drink some hot herbal tea or coffee. I don't drink it casually; I drink it fast enough to feel the warmth going down my esophagus. Once it hits my stomach, I am instantly full. This enables me to stop grazing after my meal and eliminates my desire for something sweet.

The second method I use to help with hunger and sugar cravings is drinking sparkling water. After I eat a snack or have a meal, there are times I still feel like eating. If I have a glass of sparkling water with a lemon or lime, the carbonation makes me feel full, and I can push my body away from the table to avoid over-eating.

HOW MUCH CAN YOU EAT?

People often don't know exactly how much they should eat. A good rule of thumb is to use your hand as a measuring devise. If you're wondering how much protein you should eat at a meal, lay your hand out flat, palm up. The size of your hand (including its thickness) is how much protein you should consume. For carbohydrates, make a fist. The size of your fist is the amount of low GI carbohydrates you can have on your plate. The rest of your plate can be filled with greens or vegetables.

WHERE CAN YOU EAT?

You can eat almost anywhere...Breakfast Restaurants, Chinese, Continental, Italian, Mexican, Seafood, Sushi. But remember, plan ahead, know healthy food choices, and keep the proper mindset.

Breakfast at Restaurants

Order an egg-white omelet and add any veggies you may like: onions, mushrooms, spinach, tomatoes, etc. Make sure you tell them NOT to use any butter or oil and to use non-fat cooking spray. You may use hot sauce, Pico de Gallo, or picante sauce to add flavor. You may want to order a side of oatmeal, grits or a piece of whole wheat toast without butter.

Mexican Restaurants:

Order shrimp, fish or skinless chicken breast fajitas without any oil or butter. Choose the corn tortillas (2) and flavor with Pico de Gallo, salsa, onions, a spoonful of pinto beans and a slice of avocado.

Another option is to order shrimp, fish or skinless chicken breast with Mexican spices grilled without the oil or butter. Ask your server to place those items on a bed of lettuce or with a side of steamed veggies; add salsa or Pico de Gallo for added flavor or as a dressing. If you opt out of the corn tortillas, and you are craving chips, ask your server to bring "baked" chips. A handful (5-6) of baked chips is equivalent to one corn tortilla.

If you enjoy salads, order a salad with grilled shrimp, or chicken or fish. Ask for no cheese and use Pico de Gallo or picante sauce for the dressing.

Seafood Restaurants

For starters, you can order Ceviche or Shrimp Cocktail with steamed veggies on the side without butter or oil. Another option is to order low fat fish, scallops, and shrimp and grill it in a blackened seasoning without oil or butter. Order a side of steamed veggies. If you're really hungry, order a small plain baked potato and add salsa, Pico de Gallo or ketchup for flavoring.

If you enjoy salads, order a salad with grilled salmon, scallops, shrimp or chicken. Ask for no cheese and order a fat-free dressing on the side.

Chinese Restaurant

Order steamed chicken breast, shrimp, or scallops with steamed vegetables and steamed rice. Ask the server to bring you ginger sauce, plum sauce or Lite Soy Sauce on the side to add flavor. You can also add chili pepper flakes, white pepper, and hot mustard. If you are sensitive to MSG, ask the server to prepare your food without it.

Continental Restaurants

Order a grilled skinless chicken breast, fish or shrimp seasoned with a side of steamed vegetables without oil or butter. You may also put the grilled meat on a bed of spinach and use fat free dressing, Balsamic Vinegar or salsa with garlic as a dressing. Order a plain baked or sweet potato on the side to complete the meal. Make sure you tell the server no butter or oil on the food. You can dress up the potato with salsa, ketchup, chives, pepper or fat free dressings.

If you enjoy salads, order a salad with grilled salmon, scallops, shrimp or chicken. Ask for no cheese and order a fat-free dressing on the side.

Another option is to order a grilled, skinless chicken breast or fish smothered with steamed spinach topped with tomato and onions with a side of steamed vegetables with no butter or oil. This is fantastic with garlic!

Italian Restaurants

Order grilled fish or skinless chicken breast without any sauce, butter or oil. Ask the server to bring tomato sauce or marinara sauce on the side. Order steamed vegetables without the butter or oil. Pour the sauce over the meat and vegetables and ask for fresh garlic.

If you enjoy salads, order a salad with grilled salmon, scallops, shrimp or chicken. Ask for no cheese and order a fat-free dressing on the side.

Another option is to order grilled fish or chicken with no oil or butter smothered with steamed spinach topped with tomato sauce or marinara sauce and garlic. Order steamed vegetables on the side with no oil or butter. Yummy!!

Sushi

Order tuna, snapper, scallops, shrimp, crab, or and any other low fat seafood choices on the menu. Dip it into lite soy sauce and wasabi. It is best to have these items as sashimi. This eliminates excess rice. A couple of pieces of sushi are ok.

Another option is to order the California Rolls using low fat seafood and no mayo or sauces. There are all kinds of great combinations to choose from.

WHAT IF YOU BLOW IT?

The bad news is, you blew it. The good news is you can get right back on track at the next meal or snack. Don't obsess over it and blow it for the rest of the day. That was ONLY one meal. Drop the guilt and move forward with good decisions at your next meal or snack. You don't have to eat perfectly to reap the benefits of eating healthy. If you can eat healthy at least 80% to 90% of the time you will yield HUGE results! Don't get caught up with the small stuff. Do your best and in time you will notice how easy it is to eat right for your health.

KEY POINTS:

- Know what you are going to order before you walk into the restaurant.
- Anticipate all possible obstacles before you get there.
- Do not open the menu. This gives the server a clear message that you are ordering off the menu.
- To help with your will-power, drink a "hot" beverage to decrease your hunger and help with sweet cravings.

- Remember to use your palm, and your fist as a guide when deciding how much you can eat at a meal.

- If you blow it... no worries. Focus on how you're going to make better choices at the next meal or snack.

CHAPTER FIVE

WHAT ABOUT AIRPORTS and HOTELS?

Frequent travelers know all too well what it's like to spend hours in airports, on planes, and seemingly endless nights and weeks in hotels, and at conferences. If you feel like you're always on-the-go, you know how difficult it can be to make healthy eating choices in each of these places. But you *can* succeed!

AT THE AIRPORT

The airport seems like an impossible place to find something healthy to eat. Consider Mr. Kym, the owner of a large court reporter business and a frequent flyer who complains that traveling is his worst enemy when trying to eat healthy. His day begins like this: race to the airport, get through security, run to the gate, board the plane, have a snack and something to drink. By the time he gets off the plane he is starving. It takes only a minute to smell the pizza in the food court. At this point, he knows the pizza will make him feel horrible, but he doesn't care! All good eating habits fall to the wayside and he eats whatever he can get his hands on. Unfortunately, this is a common theme among frequent flyers. Is there an alternative? After many discussions with Mr. Kym, we created a framework to help him beat this enemy, and within a couple weeks, he felt much better and even lost weight with his hectic 60 hour weeks.

I've researched the top 20 airports in the United States and have found many good places to eat. It's really very easy once you know what to look for.

Before leaving the house, there are a couple of things you can do to make your meals or snacks at the airport more manageable. Try to **plan**, **prepare** and **pack** prior to leaving for your trip. The tips on Preparing, outlined in Chapter Three, should help make your trip more successful, but there are some specifics to consider on Planning and Packing for your time at the airport and on the plane.

Planning

When making reservations, see if a meal is included on your flight. If there is, request a high protein meal or a diabetic meal. These meals are better balanced with proteins and carbohydrates compared to the high carbohydrate meal they usually serve. Consuming higher protein meals will keep you from having that spike in your blood sugar after you eat.

Stop by the grocery store and pick up some healthy food ~~that~~ to take on the plane. By having snacks available, your blood sugar won't dip too low and you'll avoid fatigue and cravings! (Make sure these snacks are on the Dr. Roxanne approved Food List.)

Packing

When packing, think about how long you'll be in the airport and on the plane. This will determine how many snacks you need to carry on the plane. Grab some fruit and several baggies of nuts and protein powder. Take a carry-on piece of luggage and pack your snacks into it. Pack your fruit, nuts and other items you want to take on the trip. Don't forget your shaker cup! A protein shake is a very convenient snack to make while eating-on-the-go. It will provide some stability in your blood sugar until you can have a healthy meal.

Again, by keeping your blood sugar balanced, you will not overeat or develop an intense craving for sugar or unhealthy carbohydrates! Pack the remainder of food in your suitcase for the duration of your trip and for the flight back home. If you have specialty items you want to pack (almond milk, Kashi *GOLEAN* cereal or tuna lunch kits), wrap them up in trash bags individually and pack them in your suitcase. This will alleviate any hassle of finding these items when you get to your destination.

What are Good Snack Choices at the Airport?

You don't have time to plan, prepare and pack? No big deal. You can still find ways to make eating-on-the-go successful while in an airport. When you arrive, go to a Newsstand or a Book Store. Typically all of these places sell snacks you can take with you on the plane. My suggestion is to find some natural nuts (almonds, walnuts or pecans), nonfat Greek yogurt or a high protein-low carbohydrate protein bar.

I'm not a big fan of protein bars. Most of them have the same amount of sugar in them as a candy bar. Look at the label. If the "total carbohydrates" are more than 20g, I would stay away from it. Look for a bar that has less than 15g of "total carbohydrates." The same theory applies for the yogurt - most have over 18g of sugar. So, for that tiny amount of yogurt there is almost 5 tsp of sugar in it. That's a lot of sugar for that tiny container of yogurt! Not only will this cause a spike in your blood sugar but it will also leave you feeling tired and fatigue within a couple of hours. Make sure your snacks are low in "total carbohydrates" and "grams of sugar."

When it's time to eat, if you don't have protein powder with you, eat half of the protein bar and a handful of nuts. If you still can't get to a healthy meal within 2 hours, have the other half of the protein bar and another handful of nuts. This should satisfy you until you can eat a healthy meal. If you found some low sugar yogurt, have a container of yogurt for your snack. **Drink plenty of water!** Traveling on airplanes has a tendency to dehydrate you. Start drinking plenty of water now so you aren't affected by this later on in your trip.

What can You Eat at the Airport?

If you have time before you board the plane, find something healthy to eat. If you are not very hungry, one thing you can do to ensure you are eating frequently is to order a meal and eat half of it now and then wait a couple of hours and eat the other half later for a snack on the plane. When deciding on what to eat at the airport... look at Chapters 3 and 4 for suggestions.

What do You Eat on the Plane?

You've finally boarded the plane. Now what? Here are some airplane tips:

- When boarding the plane, determine the last time you ate. This will give you a time frame for when you need to eat again.

- If the flight serves a meal, hopefully you requested a high protein, low carb meal in advance. This will ensure that your meal is a low GI meal. If you didn't have time to preorder your meal, try to make the meal as balanced as you can. If offered a sandwich, take the top piece of bread off to decrease the carbohydrate load. If they bring you chicken, veggies and rice... eat all of the chicken and veggies and eat a minimal amount of the starch on your plate. If they serve you a pasta dish, eat a small amount. The high amount of carbohydrates will make you feel sluggish in about an hour. A better option here would be to make a protein drink. Remember we want to keep your blood sugar balanced. By doing this, you will have more energy and prevent unwanted insulin spikes.

·   The snacks served on airplanes usually are high GI snacks. Some flights do serve peanuts, but be careful - some are honey roasted which means they have sugar.

·   If it's a long flight, after your meal, check the time so you'll know when you should have a snack. Again this might seem redundant, but you will feel much better, I promise.

·   Once you depart the plane, remember when you last ate and make a conscious effort to get in another low GI meal. For advice on what to eat, look at Chapters 3 and 4 for fast food or restaurant suggestions.

Eating-on-the-go at the airport is not difficult when you know what your options are in advance. If you plan ahead, it will make your airport decisions much easier. If you're not a planner, there are still ways to make your eating-on-the-go experiences successful. By keeping your blood sugar balanced throughout your trip, you will have more energy and decrease the chances of developing chronic illnesses due to insulin fluctuations.

AT A HOTEL

One of the biggest complaints I hear from people who spend at least 10-12 days a month in different hotels is that they have no idea how to eat-on-the-go while living the hotel life. Meet Andy, a salesman of a major corporation. A big part of his job is traveling from place to place finalizing contracts and checking on different clients. His hotel stays range from 6 to 10 times a month and he gained over 50 lbs in the last year. His biggest obstacle was eating-on-the-go while staying at different hotels. Concerned because his doctor was going to put him on cholesterol lowering medication if he didn't get a handle on his situation, he worked with me and implemented some of the strategies in this book. Andy lost 50 lbs over the next six months once he understood the guidelines of hotel eating.

Living the hotel life does not have to impede your health if you follow the basic guidelines in Chapter Three. As always, try to **plan**, **prepare** and **pack** prior to leaving for your trip.

What do You Eat at a Conference?

Most conferences will provide meals for the attendees. For some reason, when meals are provided, many people think, "It is free…I might as well eat GOOD!" Don't engage in this type of thinking! If you eat a high carbohydrate, high sugar food… your blood sugar will spike leaving you feeling tired and fatigued. These spikes and drops in your blood sugar throughout the day also can lead to weight gain and chronic illnesses. Here are some suggestions:

BREAKFAST

1. Make sure you find a protein source to eat. Most breakfast buffets have either scrambled eggs or boiled eggs. If the buffet has an omelet section, ask for an egg white omelet with any veggies you like. Request that it be cooked in nonfat cooking spray instead of butter. Protein is extremely important to have at breakfast because it maintains optimal blood sugar levels so you won't crash or feel hungry again in an hour.

2. If there is oatmeal available, have a small cup of oatmeal. Stay away from the breads.

3. Look at the fruit available. Choose 1/2 cup of the fruit from the Dr. Roxanne's approved Food List.

4. Drink a hot beverage (hot tea or coffee) to make the meal feel complete.

5. Don't forget to follow the portion sizes discussed in Chapter Two.

SNACKS

1. Sometimes the hotel will provide snacks at the conference. Usually they will lay out cookies and pastries. Stay away from these snacks! If they are too tempting, have a 1/2 of a cookie and eat a handful of almonds or walnuts.

2. If the hotel provides fruit at the break, again only eat about 1/2 cup of the fruit and eat a handful of almonds or walnuts to prevent a spike in your blood sugar.

3. It is a good idea to bring nuts or a protein drink to the conference just in case the hotel does not provide a snack.

LUNCH/DINNER

Usually lunches and dinners are served in a buffet style. This should make it easy for you to make a healthy decision. Here are some suggestions:

1. If you like salads, fill up half your plate with green leafy vegetables. Look at the different toppings and place them on the salad. Stay away from the cheeses. If you are a cheese lover, go ahead and sprinkle a LITTLE bit of cheese on your salad.

2. Don't worry about the dressing yet. Usually the vegetables and the entre are embedded in a sauce. If it's ok that your food touches, put the entre and vegetables directly on your salad. There is no need for a dressing. The sauce from the entre and vegetables will serve as the dressing.

3. IF you are someone who does NOT want their entrée and vegetables on top of their salad, then carefully look for a low-fat dressing.

4. Remember portion control. Refer to Chapter Two for details on how much protein, vegetables and carbohydrates you can have on your plate. Have larger amounts of protein and veggies. Keep any grains or starches at a minimum.

5. If bread is offered, you have a decision to make. You do not want to over-eat on starches and grains. These foods typically cause a spike in your blood sugar levels. You need to decide if you want a piece of bread, or the starchy potatoes on the buffet or the yummy dessert. Remember the portion size for a carbohy-

drate is the size of your fist. Select which one you want, and avoid the others.

6. After your meal, have a hot beverage. This will diminish the desire to go back for seconds or want a big dessert.

7. There will always be a dessert table. If you are focused on having a dessert, make sure that your meal was mostly protein and veggies. Stay away from the starches and grains. You can treat your dessert as the starch or grain.

COCKTAIL HOUR:

I don't want to spoil your fun but know this…there are approximately 20 tsp. of sugar in 12 oz. of wine; 20 tsp. of sugar in 3 shots of liquor and 20 tsp. of sugar in three beers based on the conversion of alcohol sugar to table sugar. Remember that one tsp of sugar is equivalent to one sugar packet. So 20 tsp. of sugar = 20 sugar packets! That's a lot of sugar! (Note: There is no sugar found in alcohol, only alcohol sugar which is high in calories.)

It's ok to have an adult beverage. Just understand how much sugar you are consuming. Drink in moderation. If you are watching your weight, you might want to watch your alcohol consumption.

KEY POINTS:

- Plan ahead. Go to the grocery store and get some Dr. Roxanne approved snacks for the trip. This will ensure that you have food available to snack on at the appropriate times.

- Take enough snacks with you in a carry-on. Pack the remainder of food items in your suitcase, taking enough to last the entire trip.

- When making your flight reservations, if a meal will be served on the plane, request a high protein or diabetic meal.

- If you didn't have time to plan or prepare, stop at a gift shop or newsstand prior to boarding the plan and get some Dr. Roxanne approved snack items.

- Follow the guidelines in Chapter Four to determine what to eat at restaurants

- Drink plenty of water! Traveling tends to cause dehydration.

- Alcohol is high in sugar. When trying to lose weight or gain health, drink in moderation.

CHAPTER SIX

SHOULD YOU TAKE A MULTI-VITAMIN?

If you're always on-the-go, it's a good idea to take supplements to maintain your overall health. Traveling causes an increase load on your body. This added stress strains your immune system which increases your chances of getting sick. In addition, the amount of people you come into contact with while traveling is enormous! And, unfortunately, many of these people travel sick or are carrying a virus from a sick family member. With increased stress and a strained immune system, it's only a matter of time before you get sick. By taking supplements, you can increase your total health and support your immune system so you will stay healthy year round.

Many people believe that if they eat healthy they don't need to supplement their diets. This is so far from the truth.

Our soil is more depleted of vitamins and minerals than ever before. Many fruits and vegetables are taken off the vine prematurely so that they have a nice color by the time they are delivered to the grocery stores. This depletes these foods of their natural antioxidants and vitamin status.

Antioxidants are very important to take especially when you are under the stressors of traveling – they protect the body from free radical damage. The two antioxidants I suggest you start with are Vitamin C and Greens. Vitamin C is a good antioxidant to incorporate in traveling regimen. I recommend that you take 4 – 6 grams of Vitamin C per day while you're in your traveling season. If 6 grams is too much for your stomach to tolerate then decrease your amount down to 4 grams a day. This can be divided daily into two or three dosages.

Greens is another excellent source of antioxidants. It is a powder mix loaded with certified organic, whole food plant extracts. Oxygen Radical Absorbance Capacity (ORAC) is a method of measuring antioxidant capacities of different foods. The USDA recommends ORAC unit ingestion of 3,000-5,000 ORAC units daily. Each scoop of the Greens has a high ORAC value of 20,000+ providing at least four times the USDA recommendation. I put one scoop of the powder green mix in 4 oz. of water 1-2 times a day. It is easy to travel with and the health benefits are extraordinary!

TO ENSURE PROPER NUTRIENT STATUS I RECOMMEND:

- A good multivitamin/mineral
- An additional B complex
- Fish oil (omega 3) - 2,000 to 4,000 mg/day
- Magnesium - 350 to 400 mg/day
- Vitamin D3 with K2 - 2,000 to 5,000 IU/day
- Antioxidants
- Probiotics - A combination of Bifidobacteria, Lactobacilli and Streptococci.

Note: People on medications may need additional supplementation because these drugs can deplete the body and prevent the absorption of important nutrients. For example, statin users should incorporate CoQ10 (100-200 mg) in their diets and people taking acid blockers or birth control should be taking additional B vitamins (preferably by intramuscular injections).

For a list of supplements I use in my office log on to www.DrRoxanne.com. These supplements are pharmaceutical grade; they are safe and very effective in providing support and well-being for thousands of individuals.

HOW MUCH WATER SHOULD YOU DRINK?

Drink plenty of water! Seventy-five percent of Americans are chronically dehydrated. Mild dehydration will slow down your metabolism as much as three percent. As a traveler, water is extremely important in flushing out impurities in your body. When you travel, the cabin pressure in the airplanes, the closed air circulation of hotel rooms as well as the toxic substances you are exposed to, creates a scenario for dehydration. If you don't hydrate, these impurities stay in your system longer which can lead to a compromised immune system and an overall feeling of fatigue.

How much water should you drink? A good rule of thumb is to take your body weight and divide by two. This is how many ounces of water you should be drinking daily. For instance, a 150 pound individual should consume 75 oz. of water a day. (150 pound person divided by 2 = 75 ounces)

CONCLUSION

In conclusion, eating on-the-go is a healthy lifestyle habit that is IMPORTANT to master! Many of my patients' health issues are related to poor choices made while traveling. By learning how to make better food choices, you can potentially prevent or even reverse chronic illnesses from taking control of your life!

A direct quote from the prestigious New England Journal of Medicine, 1998 states: *"Not only do persons with better health habits survive longer, but in such persons, disability is postponed and compressed into fewer years at the end of life."* Disabilities due to chronic conditions can be postponed to the last years of your life if you make better choices now! It is the lifestyle choices you make on a daily basis that will have the greatest impact on your long-term health.

Don't let this be you. Master this information so you don't become a statistic! Living longer in the absence of health and vitality is not the goal for most people. So "**add life**" to your years, not "**years**" to your life – start making better choices while eating-on-the-go!

APPENDIX

DR. ROXANNE'S APPROVED FOOD LIST

The following are foods to include in your meal plan. Remember to watch out for high fat foods which have been linked to heart disease. I've included a category for healthy fats, which have great health benefits, but be careful - too much of these fats can lead to weight gain.

PROTEINS

Try to get in 4-5 servings a day

APPROVED PROTEINS	SERVING SIZE	# OF CARBS
EGGS	1	0.6g
EGG WHITES	4-6	0-trace g
EGG SUBSTITUTE	2/3 cup	0-trace g
FISH: Cod, Halibut, Tilapia, Sea Bass, Tuna, Salmon, Orange Roughy	4-5 oz	0-trace g

TUNA: canned (water packed) or market fresh	4-5 oz	0-trace g
SHELLFISH: Lobster, Shrimp, Crab, Scallops	4-5 oz	0-trace g
CHICKEN: breast only skinless	4-5 oz	0-trace g
TURKEY: breast only skinless	4-5 oz	0-trace g
LAMB: leg or lean roast	4-5 oz	0-trace g
LEAN BEEF	4 -6 oz	0-trace g
LEAN WHITE PORK (Pork Loins, Chops, etc)	4 -6 oz	0-trace g
VEAL	4-5 oz	0-trace g
YOGURT: Plain nonfat	4 oz	6.0g
YOGURT: Greek nonfat	4 oz	7.0g
COTTAGE CHEESE: Low fat	4 oz	1.5g
CHEESE (Feta, Goat)	1 oz	1.0g
MILK: skim, rice, almond, soy	4 oz	6.0g
TOFU	½ cup	5.4 g
SEITEN	3 slices	3.0g
TEMPEH	4 oz	8.0g

<u>VEGETABLES</u>

Vegetables should be fresh or frozen – not canned.
You may eat 6-8 servings a day.

APPROVED VEGETABLES	SERVING SIZE	# OF CARBS
Asparagus	6 spears	4.0g
Artichokes	½ cup	8.0g
Sprouts	½ cup	3.1g
Bell Peppers	1 small	3.5g
Broccoli	½ cup	5.0g
Cauliflower	½ cup	3.5
Celery	1 stalk 7.5in	1.5g
Cucumber	½ cup	1.5g
Dill Pickle	1 small	1.5g
Cabbage	½ cup	2.5g
Onions, Leeks	½ onion	4.5g
Garlic	1 clove	1.0g
Chives	1 Tbsp	0.1g
Eggplant	½ cup	7.0g
Green Beans	½ cup	4.9g
Mushrooms	½ cup	4.22g
Okra	½ cup	3.5g
Radishes	2 small	.14g
Tomatoes	1 small	3.57g

Squash – Yellow, Zucchini, Spaghetti	½ cup	3.5g
Jalapeno Pepper	2 small	1.66g
Kelp	1 cup	1.0g
Greens	1 cup	3.0g
Lettuce	2 cups	2.3g
Spinach leaves	2 cup	2.18
Spinach frozen	½ cup	3.5g

GRAINS/STARCHES

It is best to have 1-3 servings a day from this category. Do not exceed 3 servings! If you're trying to lose weight, do not exceed 1-2 servings a day from this category. People with diabetes, insulin resistance, or if you struggle with stubborn abdominal fat, minimize your carbohydrates to 50-75 grams a day.

APPROVED GRAINS/STARCHES	SERVING SIZE	# OF CARBS
Rice, cooked	1/2-3/4 cup	24g-36g
Quinoa, cooked	1/2-3/4 cup	25g-35g
Potatoes- sweet, russet, red	6-8 oz	25g
Pasta- rice, spinach	3/4 cup	26g-40g
Crackers Nut-thins	8-10	12g-15g
Cereal- Kashi Go Lean	1/2 cup	15g

Cereal- Cream of rice, slow cooked oats	1/2 cup	28g
Low Carb Tortilla	1-2	5g-10g
CrispBread	1-2	7g-14g
Popcorn (popped)94% fat free	1 cup	4.6g
Corn tortilla	1 -2	11g-22g
Bread- multi grain lite	1 slice	11.4g

LEGUMES

Legumes are high in carbohydrates and need to be monitored. You can substitute beans for a starch/carb but don't consume both legumes and carbohydrates at a meal.

APPROVED LEGUMES	SERVING SIZE	# OF CARBS
Beans – Garbanzo, Pinto, Fat-free refried, Black,	1/2 cup	20-25g
Lima, Cannellini, Navy, Mung	1/2 cup	25g
Green Soy Beans - Edamame	1 cup	20g
Peas – Yellow/green split peas, Sweet green peas	1/2 cup	21g
Lentils – Red and green	1/2 cup	20g
Bean Soups – ¾ cup	3/4c	25-30g
Hummus	1/2c	18g

FRUITS

Do not exceed more than two servings of fruit a day. Although fruit is a healthy snack, it also contains fruit sugars and carbohydrates which can lead to unbalanced blood sugar levels. Be sure to follow the serving sizes.

APPROVED FRUITS	SERVING SIZE	# OF CARBS
Avocado (California)	½	6.0g
Avocado (Florida) NOT A GOOD CHOICE!	½	14g
Blackberries	½ cup	9.2g
Blueberries	½ cup	10.0g
Cantaloupe	½ cup	7.0g
Grapefruit (pink)	half	9.5g
Grapes	½ cup	8.0g
Honeydew	1/4 cup	7.7g
Lemon	1 medium	5.4g
Lemon juice, fresh	1 Tbsp	1.3g
Lime juice	1 oz	2.8g
Peach	1 small	9.7g
Rhubarb (4 oz.)	4 oz	3.5g
Strawberries	½ cup	5.5g

HEALTHY FATS

Eat only 2-3 servings a day from this category. These are healthy fats but should not be eaten in excess. Avoid honey roasted nuts.

APPROVED NUTS	SERVING SIZE	# OF CARBS
Almonds	7	1.5g
Walnuts	7	5.0g
Pecans halves	7	2.5g
Peanuts – natural	10	3.0g
Natural Nut Butter	1 tsp	3.5
Sunflower	2 tsp	3.0g
Sesame	2 tsp	3.0g
Pumpkin	2 tsp	3.0g

APPROVED OILS	SERVING SIZE	# OF CARBS
Flaxseed Oil (refrigerate)	1 tsp	0
Walnut Oil	1 tsp	0
Extra Virgin Olive Oil	1 tsp	0
Canola Oil and Sesame Oil	1 tsp	0
Olives	8-10	
Avocado	1/4 of a whole	
Butter	1 tsp	

SPICES/CONDIMENTS

There are no limitations on spices. Season your food to your taste. If you have high blood pressure, be careful with high sodium seasonings. Also, be careful with Ketchup and other condiments - they contain sugar.

APPROVED SPICES/CONDIMENTS	SERVING SIZE	# OF CARBS
Cinnamon, cumin, dill, ginger, oregano, parsley, rosemary, turmeric, thyme, etc.		0 g
Herbs		0 g
Vinegar		0 g
Lime/Lemon		0 g
Soy Sauce	1 Tbsp	2. g
Ketchup	1 Tbsp	4.0 g
Worcestershire Sauce	1 Tbsp	2.7 g

SWEETENERS

*** NOTE: Artificial sweeteners can have harmful effects on the body. Limit them!

APPROVED SWEETENERS	SERVING SIZE	# OF CARBS
Stevia		0 g
Truvia		0 g
Splenda/Equal***		0 g

BEVERAGES

*** NOTE: Coffee and other caffeinated products can cause a spike in insulin levels creating an unhealthy scenario. And diet drinks contain artificial sweeteners. BEWARE.

APPROVED BEVERAGES	SERVING SIZE	# OF CARBS
Filtered Water		0 g
Seltzer/Mineral Water		0 g
Herbal Teas		0 g
Tea – green, white, black		0 g
Coffee ***		0 g
Decaffeinated Coffee		0 g
Diet Soda (limit one per day)***		0 g
Calorie Free Drink		0 g

FOODS TO AVOID
Consume in Moderation

PROTEINS:	GRAINS/STARCHES:
Cheeses	Processed Cereals
Red Meat	White bread
Chicken Thighs	Crackers
Turkey Thighs	Chips
Pork	
Cold Cuts	LEGUMES:
Deli Meat	Canned beans
Sausage	Canned Peas
Hot Dogs	
All other Pork products (bacon, sausage, etc)	FRUITS:
Whole Milk	Fruit Juices
Yogurt with fruit	Dried Fruit
	Bananas
VEGETABLES:	Figs
Corn	Prunes
Creamed Veggies	
Veggies w/cheese	
Veggies in sauces	

FATS AND OILS:	NUTS AND SEEDS:
Shortening	Honey Roasted
Processed Oil	Trail mix
Hydrogenated Oils	nuts that contains added oils
CONDIMENTS USE SPARINGLY:	BEVERAGES:
Ketchup	Soft Drinks
bbq Sauce	Gatorade
Mayo	PowerAde
Other condiments	Energy Drinks
	Sweetened Beverage
SWEETENERS:	Alcohol
Refined Sugar	
Syrups	
Fruit or Plant Sugar	

FOOD JOURNAL
Eating-On-The-Go

MONDAY	TIME	DESCRIPTION	DATE
Wake Time:			
Breakfast			
Snack			
Lunch			
Snack			
Dinner			
Water (ounces)			
Other Drinks			
Sleep Time:			

Made in the USA
Monee, IL
18 August 2022

11858389R00050